KISS

KISS

A HEALTH GUIDE FOR PEOPLE WHO LIKE TO KEEP IT SIMPLE

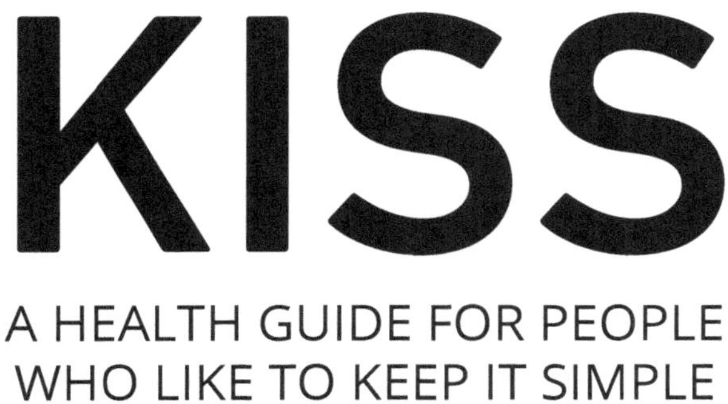

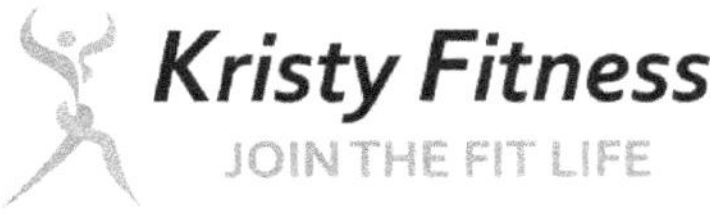

KRISTY BUSSARD

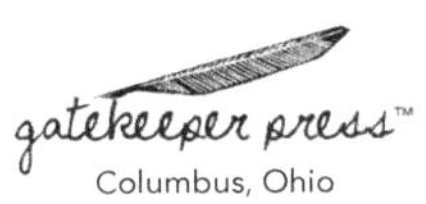

KISS: A Health Guide for People
Who Like to Keep it Simple

Published by Gatekeeper Press
2167 Stringtown Rd, Suite 109
Columbus, OH 43123-2989
www.GatekeeperPress.com

Library of Congress Control Number: 2021941462

ISBN (paperback): 9781662914430
eISBN: 9781662914447

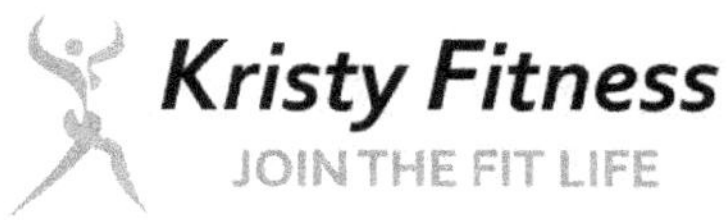

Contents

Keep **I**t **S**imple **S**illy vii

The 80/20 Rule xi

Simple vs Easy xv

LIFE-CHANGING STEPS 1

STEP ONE: Eliminate The Non-Negotiables
From Your Diet 3

STEP TWO: Eat Only Whole Foods 11

STEP THREE: Movement............................. 15

STEP FOUR: Eliminate Stressful People,
Places, And Things...................................... 19

STEP FIVE: Set Goals 21

STEP SIX: Get Accountability....................... 23

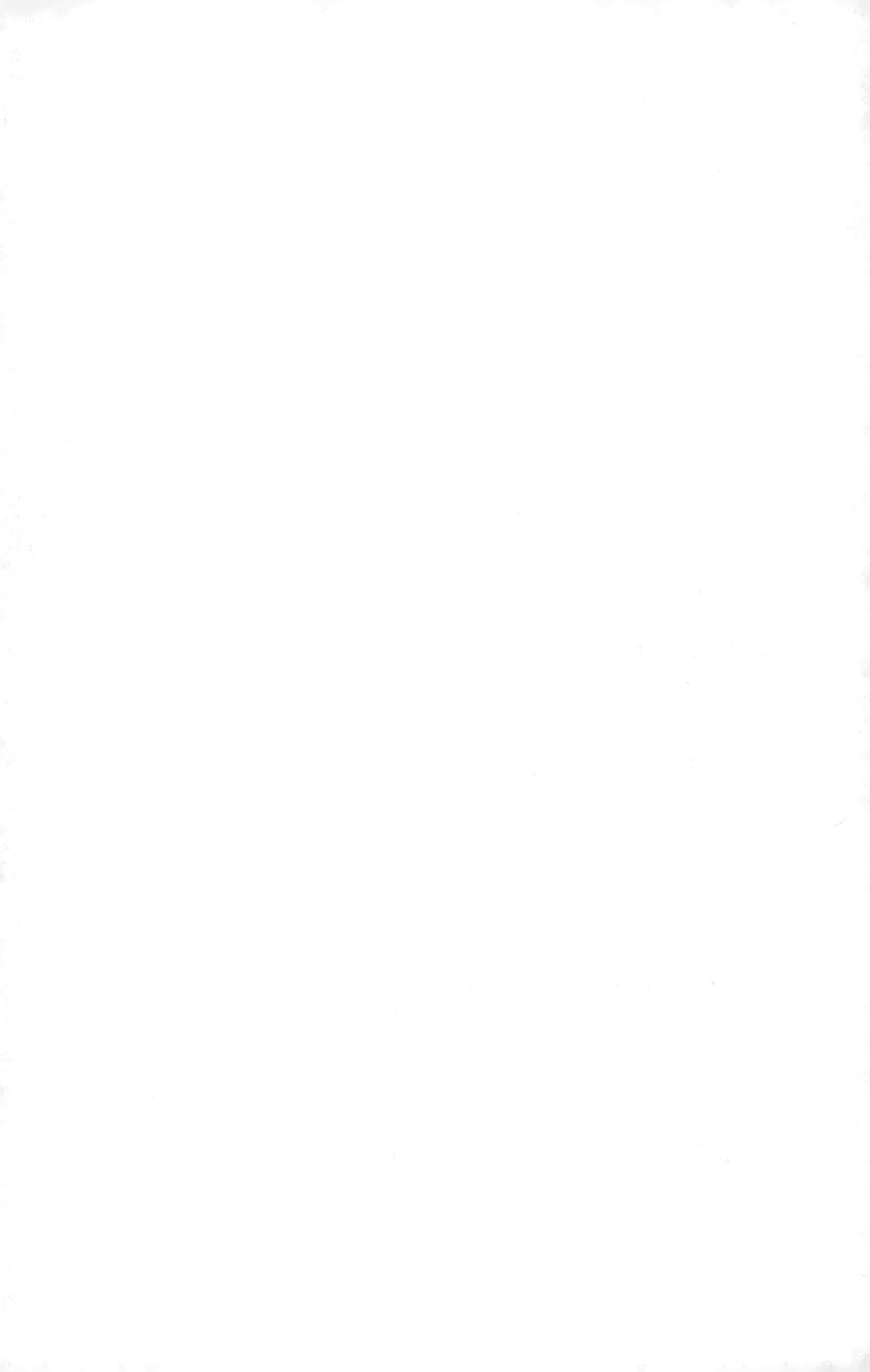

Keep **I**t **S**imple **S**illy

KISS THOSE SYMPTOMS GOODBYE!

A HEALTH GUIDE FOR PEOPLE WHO LIKE TO KEEP THINGS SIMPLE

- Do you wish you had a leaner, more toned body?

- Do you have a really hard time losing weight?

- Do you feel tired all the time and find yourself drinking caffeine just to function?

- Do you feel like you have brain fog and little clarity?

- Do your muscles ache and joints hurt for no apparent reason?

- Do you have digestive issues like gas and bloating, or constipation/diarrhea?

- Do you have trouble sleeping through the night or at all?

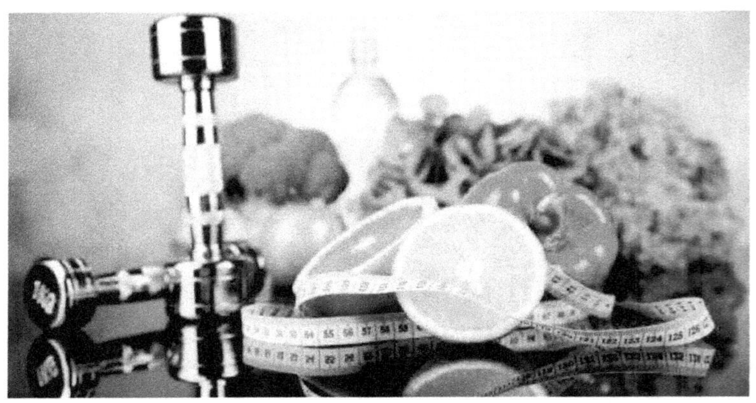

SYMPTOMS OF TOXICITY

Why am I starting this guide with a bunch of questions? Because these questions are your symptoms! If I told you that I am a health practitioner who can help you make some lifestyle changes to get rid of these symptoms, you might not understand what that means. You would probably not even associate some of these issues with lifestyle choices. You would likely go to a medical doctor, thinking a pill might fix it. (Good luck with that!) This guide is full of some very simple, practical solutions on how to reduce these negative issues and symptoms from your body and life. This is not rocket science! This is just pure and simple information that will change your life. If you are like me, you don't want some complicated book where you have to read 500 pages, and half of it you instantly forget. You just want someone to get right to the point on what to do to help.

The 80/20 Rule

Have you ever heard of the 80/20 Principle? Also known as the Pareto Principle, it is an aphorism which asserts that 80 percent of outcomes (or outputs) result from 20 percent of causes (or inputs) for any given event.

This is a great way to start this simple guide to taking you from a place with all or some of these symptoms I already mentioned, to a place of being symptom-free, or at the very least 80 percent symptom-free. (The other 20 percent we will need to discuss a little deeper, but that is down the road.)

This principle can be applied in so many ways, but I want to refer to it from a place of experience. In my 20 years as a Wellness Practitioner (helping people change their lives by making necessary food and lifestyle changes), **I can definitely say that all my clients and patients who have followed this SIMPLE way of life have experienced at least an 80 percent reduction in their symptoms that they came to me to get help for.** I think it is wise for someone to take a moment and consider if they really want to use the word "heal," even an MD or other physician. I say this because the original job of medicine was referred to as a "practice." This means that patient and physician will practice a method until there is symptom reduction (that is, the appearance of being healed, as long as they continue the practice). If the symptom is just deadened by a chemical substance like medicine, then there is no healing at all, just the elimination of the signal telling the person that something is wrong. I practice Functional Wellness, which means I identify symptoms that reveal where to start with a patient, and then I educate the patient on how to practice with me until they are well (by which I mean symptom-free). Again, they will be symptom-free as long as they practice the methods that made the change to help the body reduce symptoms.

PLEASE KEEP IN MIND THAT THIS IS A GUIDE TO HELP A PERSON REDUCE THESE SYMPTOMS OVER A PERIOD OF TIME (IF THEY ACTUALLY DO WHAT IS SUGGESTED). SOME WILL BE SYMPTOM-FREE SOONER THAN OTHERS, BECAUSE EACH SUGGESTION I MAKE LEADS THE PERSON'S BODY TO A PLACE OF BEING LESS TOXIC. IT IS CELLULAR TOXICITY THAT LEADS TO THESE AILMENTS THAT PLAGUE OUR BODIES. WHAT I TELL PEOPLE IS: "YOU ARE BEGINNING A DETOX TO GOOD HEALTH." A HEALTHY BODY IS A LEAN, FOCUSED, HIGHLY ENERGIZED BODY. IT TAKES SOME LONGER TO DETOX THAN OTHERS; BUT IF YOU STICK IT OUT, MOST PEOPLE WILL FIRST SEE RESULTS WITHIN 2 TO 12 WEEKS. THIS IS NOT A CRASH DIET, SO TO EXPECT RESULTS IMMEDIATELY IS UNREALISTIC. IT IS A JOURNEY, NOT AN INSTANT FIX. IT BECOMES A LIFESTYLE. YOU GET BETTER AND BETTER ONE DAY AT A TIME, AND IT BECOMES CONTAGIOUS. YOUR FRIENDS WILL WANT WHAT YOU HAVE! FUNNY THING IS, WHEN YOU TELL THEM HOW SIMPLE THIS IS, THEY MIGHT NOT EVEN BELIEVE YOU!

Simple vs Easy

NOW REMEMBER: I said simple, not easy. 'Simple' is something that is not complicated at all. 'Easy' is something that does not take much effort. This will take some effort for some of you. Anything worth having is going to involve effort. The discipline you use to get the benefits of this program will also boost your self-confidence, and help you go on to achieve the next amazing thing in your life! I see that ALL THE TIME!

LIFE-CHANGING STEPS

HERE ARE YOUR SIMPLE STEPS NEEDED TO CHANGE YOUR LIFE AND BE HEALTHY!

Eliminate The Non-Negotiables From Your Diet

When discussing possible dietary changes a patient can make to bring healing to the body, we always have a discussion about the "non-negotiables," the big three being processed wheat, dairy, and processed sugar. This is a term I learned during my training that has to do with the fact that most people who are suffering from any kind of digestion issues (or even autoimmune disorders) need to consider if they are willing to give up these three processed food groups. By the way, 80 percent of patients who give up these foods for 90 days or more no longer have any noticeable symptoms.

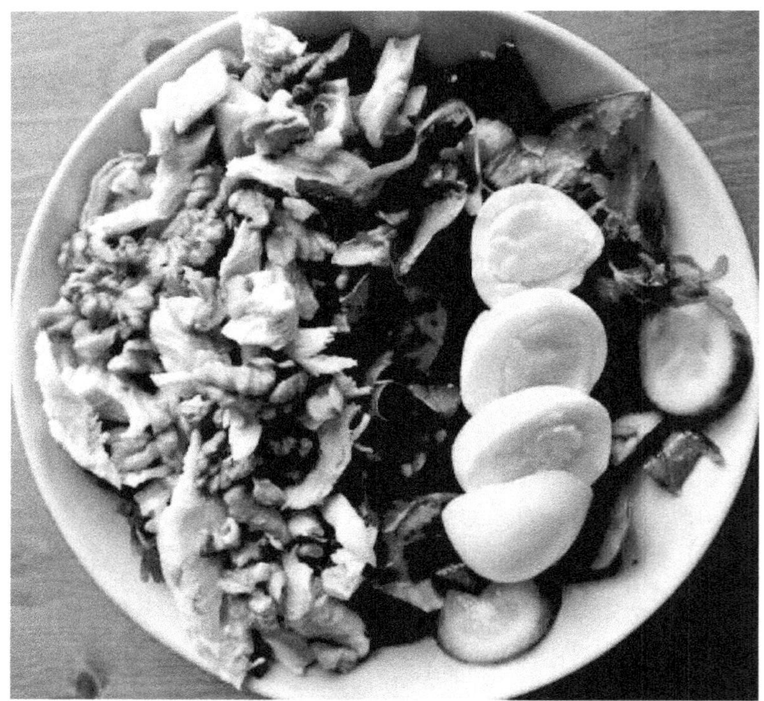

Why is processed wheat considered a "non-negotiable?"

In the 1870s, the invention of modern steel roller mills revolutionized grain milling. Compared to old stone methods, it was fast and efficient and gave fine control over the various parts of the kernel. Instead of just mashing it all together, one could separate (or "process") the component parts, allowing the purest and finest of white flour to be easily produced at low cost.

And, beyond being cheap and wildly popular, this new type of flour shipped and stored better, allowing for a long distribution chain. In fact, it keeps almost indefinitely.

Pest problems were eliminated because pests do not want it. Of course, we now know that the reason it keeps so well is that it has been stripped of vital nutrients.

The steel roller mill became so popular so fast that within 10 years nearly all stone mills in the Western world had been replaced. And thus was born the first "processed food" and the beginning of our industrial food system: where vast quantities of shelf-stable "food" are produced in large factories, many months and many miles from the point of consumption.

This excerpt from Wikipedia says it well: "From a human nutrition standpoint, it is ironic that wheat milling methods to produce white flour eliminate those portions of the wheat kernel (bran, germ, shorts, and red dog mill streams) that are richest in proteins, vitamins, lipids and minerals."

While these "advances" in milling were hailed as an innovation of modern living, nobody thought much about what was happening to the actual food value of wheat. It was now an unhealthy "food" causing havoc on the digestive system.

Why is dairy considered a "non-negotiable?"

Pasteurization was first introduced in the late 1800s. It was first applied to dairy products after the spread of numerous milk-borne infections in the population. It refers to the heating of milk to a temperature higher than the boiling point, and then rapidly cooling it.

This process supposedly removes the bacteria and other harmful particles found in conventionally produced milk. However, pasteurization renders essential enzymes and nutrients inactive. Without these essential enzymes, our bodies cannot effectively digest it.

Although pasteurized milk is strongly recommended and advertised by both the CDC and FDA, its safety is questionable. While raw milk enthusiasts are commonly lambasted because they supposedly "expose themselves to a higher risk of milk-borne bacteria," pasteurized milk consumers have a higher chance of ingesting chemicals and other toxins from conventional dairy factories.

Because of pasteurization and other filtering processes, factory milk producers commonly raise cows in unhealthy, cramped environments, where they are fed an unnatural diet of grains and corn. This is mainly because they are dependent on pasteurization's ability to kill off pathogens or filter antibiotics that may have leaked into their milk products.

But while they claim that this is entirely safe, the nutrient content and overall quality of these milk products is compromised. Pasteurization removes the essential nutrients and compounds that are beneficial to the human body. Studies show that this process deactivates the enzymes that are necessary for the human digestion of milk, kills off the good bacteria that may be beneficial to the human body, alters the calcium content, and removes most of the vitamin C in raw milk. Since dairy products like cheese and yogurt are made from milk, it is all considered a non-negotiable.

Why is processed sugar considered a "non-negotiable?"

Dr. Robert Lustig, a professor of clinical pediatrics in the division of endocrinology at the University of California, and a pioneer in decoding sugar metabolism, says that your body can safely metabolize up to 6 teaspoons of added sugar per day.

But since most Americans are consuming about three times that amount, most of the excess sugar gets turned into body fat, leading to the debilitating chronic metabolic diseases that many people are struggling with.

Here are some of the effects that excessive sugar intake has on your health:

- **It overloads and damages your liver.** The effects of too much sugar or fructose can be likened to the effects of alcohol. All the fructose you eat gets shuttled to the only organ that has the transporter for it: your liver.

- This severely taxes and overloads the organ, leading to potential liver damage.

- **It tricks your body into gaining weight, and affects your insulin and leptin signaling.** Sugar fools your metabolism by turning off your body's appetite control system. It fails to stimulate insulin, which in turn fails to suppress ghrelin, or "the hunger hormone." This then fails to stimulate leptin, or "the satiety hormone." This causes you to eat more and develop an even bigger resistance to insulin.

- **It causes metabolic dysfunction.** Eating too much sugar causes a barrage of symptoms known as classic metabolic syndrome. These include weight gain, abdominal obesity, decreased levels of HDL (or "good" cholesterol) and increased levels of LDL (or "bad" cholesterol), elevated blood sugar, elevated triglycerides, and high blood pressure.

- **It increases your uric acid levels.** High uric acid levels are a risk factor for heart and kidney disease. In fact, the connection between sugar, metabolic syndrome, and uric acid is now so clear that your uric acid level can effectively be used as a marker for sugar toxicity.

Eat Only Whole Foods

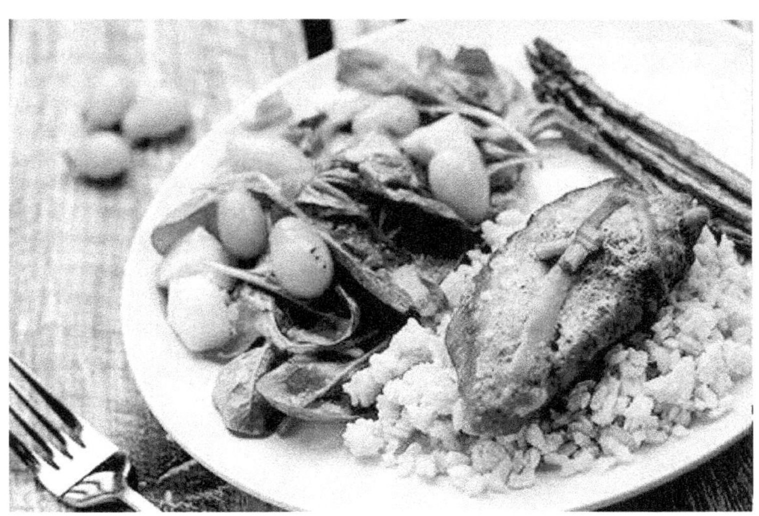

W hole foods are basically foods that are still in their original form.

Remember to eat foods "clean" (that is, without condiments, breading, smothered in butter, etc.) until you have reached your goal, whatever that might be. (I will discuss setting a goal in more detail at the end of this book.) For now, plan on eating 4 small meals 3 hours apart each day, then fasting the other 12 hours, counting backwards from when you usually wake up. (That is, if you usually wake at 6 a.m., you should begin fasting at 6 p.m.) Supplement this with as much spring or filtered water as you can drink per day, while limiting yourself to just a small amount of caffeine in the early morning.

Organic whole food (grown without pesticides or synthetic fertilizers) is best to eliminate the toxins that are in some conventional foods, but this is not essential. If you are sick and suffering, though, definitely go organic!

WHOLE FOODS LIST

Beef, chicken, and fish. Ground is fine. No nuggets, nothing deep fried, nothing breaded. CLEAN! Grill it, bake it, slow cook it. Get creative with seasonings and sauces.

Eggs. Organic is best, as is "free range," which means that the chickens are allowed to roam freely in a pasture during the day.

Old-fashioned (rolled) oats. Plain, no sugar. Absolutely no processed "oatmeal packets."

Veggies. Both raw and cooked are great. Consider substituting veggies for grain dishes, such as zucchini pasta and cauliflower rice.

Fruits. Not from a jar, tube, or other container. Just raw and fresh.

Potatoes and sweet potatoes. Baked potatoes are fine, but remember, no cheese or sour cream.

Rice. Pretty much any plain rice is good. Stay away from processed "rice dishes" in a box.

Quinoa, couscous, barley, popcorn, and other whole grains. Grains are not bad unto themselves, as long as you're eating the kind that leave in the entire kernel. A good rule of thumb is to avoid any white grains, such as white flour and white bread.

Nuts and nut butters. Raw nuts are best, although you should only have a handful with your meal or as a snack. The exception is peanuts (which are actually legumes, not technically "nuts"), which you should avoid altogether. Almond butter and other nut butters are a great substitute for peanut butter.

Clarified butter/ghee. Clarified butter (known in Southeast Asia as "ghee") is butter that has been slowly cooked so to remove everything but the pure butterfat.

Balsamic vinegar and olive oil. Great for salad dressings. As always, avoid processed salad dressings premixed in a bottle. Remember, anything with canola or soybean oil is toxic! Use olive oil in its raw form only, because once you heat it, it becomes a trans-fat, which is not good. (Instead, cook using coconut oil or grapeseed oil.)

Raw honey and stevia. A great alternative to processed sugar for sweetening foods and beverages.

Movement

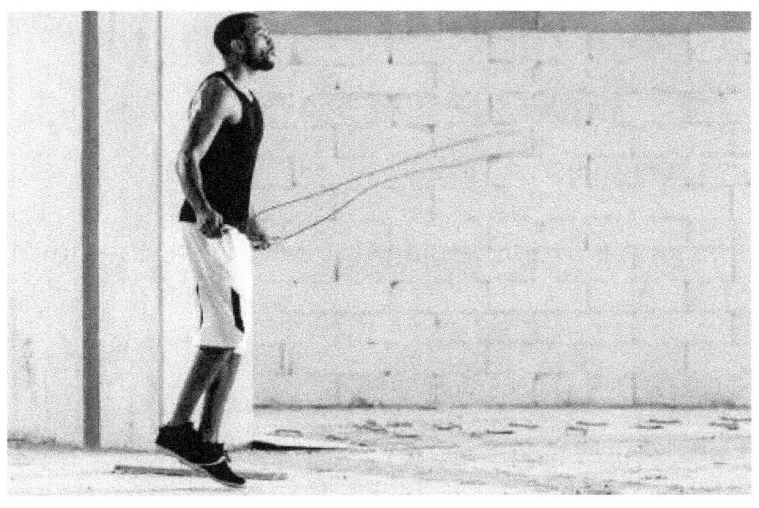

'M NOT INTO PEOPLE GOING OUT AND KILLING THEMSELVES AT RUNNING OR CROSSFIT, SO I PROVIDE A VERY SIMPLE BUT EFFECTIVE

WORKOUT INSTEAD. THIS WORKOUT WILL HELP INCREASE YOUR METABOLIC RATE AS WELL AS TONE THAT BODY.

MUSCLE TRAINING 3 DAYS A WEEK

Do 3 sets of 20 repetitions for each:

- Bicep curls with band
- Tricep curls with band
- Back squeezes with band
- Bridges/pelvic tilts

End with a 1-minute plank (or work up to 1 minute).

CARDIO 3 DAYS A WEEK

Best if done on a fasted stomach. As always, take breaks as necessary.

Begin with a cardio/power walk for 30 minutes.

End with a 1-minute plank (or work up to 1 minute).

View a demonstration video:
https://www.youtube.com/watch?v=aBFlprDu6ul

REST 1 DAY A WEEK

Very important! For emotional stress and an achy body, do this stretch and breathe routine with me. It is amazing in so many ways. Great to do before bed every night of the week, not just your rest day. Video: https://youtu.be/0xoQP_kbDak

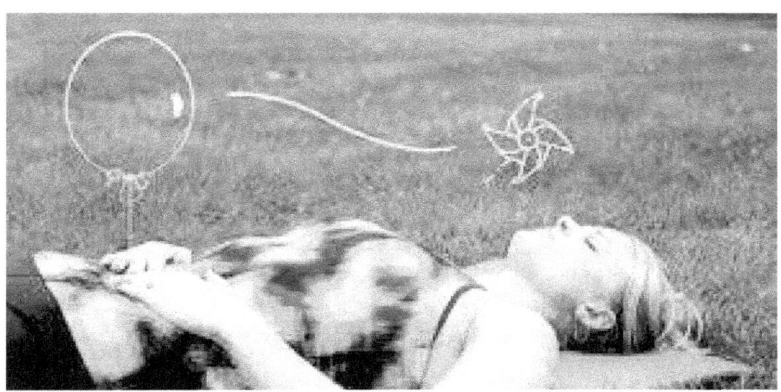

Eliminate Stressful People, Places, And Things

One of the last things to discuss is detoxing stress from the body. All the symptoms I mentioned in the beginning of this guide are usually an indication of adrenal stress or even complete adrenal failure. I recommend eliminating any stressful people and/or situations in your life as much as you reasonably can. You know who and what they are.

I also recommend finding time in each day to mentally decompress, and reach a place of calm and quiet. I myself, for example, am a big believer in prayer, while other people might prefer meditation, a gratitude journal, mindfulness exercises, or a leisurely walk around their neighborhood.

Set Goals

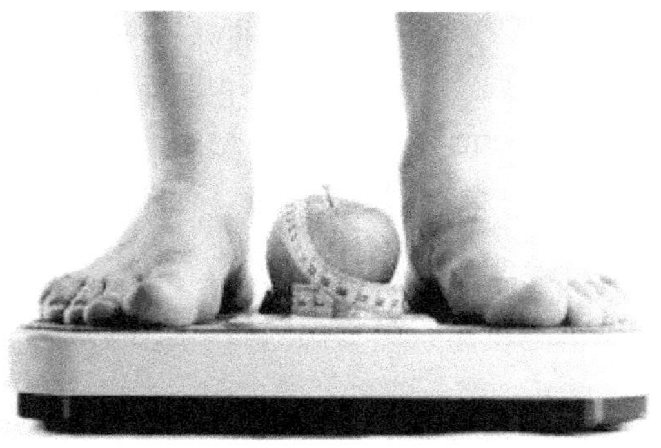

Set a goal for yourself. If your main issue is weight loss resistance, then pick a weight you would like to be and don't stop until you get there. Eventually this will become your lifestyle, and you will learn how to incorporate cheat meals and even cheat drinks without going back to a toxic place.

Maybe you want to reduce the digestive issues you have each day. Continue until you reach that goal, and then learn to incorporate cheat meals on occasion. The same goes for any symptoms you want to reduce, but DO NOT GO BACK TO THE OLD LIFESTYLE. Remember: We practice wellness, which means continuing to practice one day at a time until you are a new you, living a new lifestyle. Free from pain, fatigue, and brain fog...FOREVER!

Get Accountability

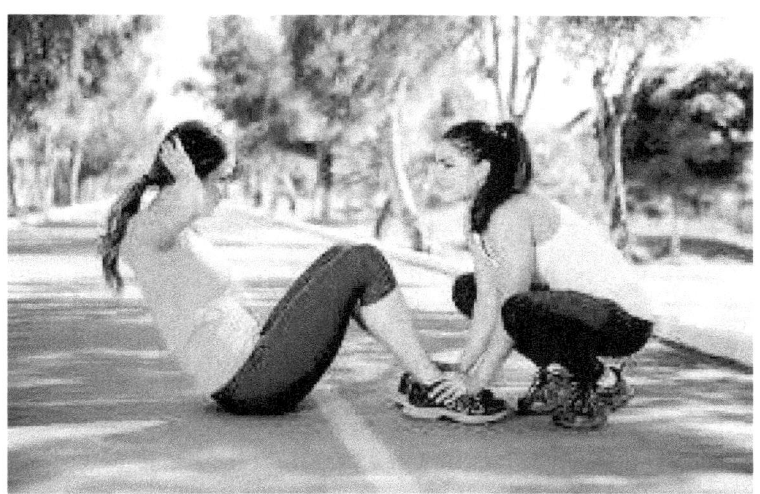

nvite a friend to do this with you. One of the biggest reasons why people fail at these "get healthy" attempts is because they have no accountability. **If you and a friend, or small group, commit to do this together, you will succeed.** Just make sure you invite those friends who will be real with you, not just nice! My best friends are the ones who tell me what I *need* to hear, not what I *want* to hear. Remember to be honest about those stressful people and things you need to get rid of. You will want to have your friends know about these stressful things as well, so be open. That is how accountability works. Post your goal on Facebook or Instagram, or tell a bunch of friends, and take that 'before' pic. These are also all great ways to be accountable.

And please remember one last thing, which is that you can ask me any questions you might have at @KristyBFitness on Facebook. I'm happy to describe what a "small meal" looks like. I will send out recipe ideas. I will do whatever I can to help you succeed! I will walk this journey with you as much as I can.

Remember, this is simple, so do not complicate it! Just eat real whole foods, exercise regularly, and detox emotionally.

If you'd like to join a larger community of readers who are all going through this journey with you, please post your name and story on my KristyBFitness Facebook page. And please post your 'after' pictures! Those are so encouraging! I am praying for you!